# FIRE, FAITH & GLORY

*Le Feu, La Foi et La Gloire*

R.R.Pravin

authorHOUSE®

*AuthorHouse™*
*1663 Liberty Drive*
*Bloomington, IN 47403*
*www.authorhouse.com*
*Phone: 1 (800) 839-8640*

*Published by AuthorHouse  08/09/2018*

*ISBN: 978-1-5462-5480-5 (sc)*
*ISBN: 978-1-5462-5481-2 (hc)*
*ISBN: 978-1-5462-5479-9 (e)*

Dedicated to all of us who are hoping for a better tomorrow for the children we work with everyday & their families, & to all the children who have taught me that life is worth living to the fullest each and every day.

*Dédié à tous les enfants et leurs familles qui restent toujours nos inspirations. C'est grâce à vous qu'on a eu l'occasion d'améliorer l'humanité et apprendre que des miracles existent toujours. Il ne faut jamais perdre l'espoir.*

# CONTENTS

# FOREWORD BY A PAEDIATRIC INTENSIVIST

The intensive care unit is a place where patients' (and their family's) emotions frequently run amok with anger, denial, sadness, guilt and grief. It is a place where positive news is broken with liberating relief, or negative news is broken with anguish, burning tears and crushing heartache. This is where I work and try to keep sanity in the unit. Paediatric residents do postings with us to expose them to the breath of critical illness in children.

Pravin joined the paediatric residency program in KK Women's and Children's Hospital, Singapore, in 2016. He is frequently referred to as the resident who has a keen interest in paediatric palliative care. In fact, he made an impression on me the first day we met. I recall we were covering the high dependency unit, a ward for moderately ill children, some of whom may have impending need for intensive care. One patient had a complex cardiac disease for which his family had opted not for surgical correction as the surgical risk was unacceptably high. This child, now nearly a teenager was reaching end stage disease. Even after all these years, his family found it hard to come to terms with the end. At this point, having forgone the surgery in earlier stages of the disease, there was no cure. "Death" a natural part of "life" was inevitably approaching. Offering invasive life support was not going to reverse the disease and most likely will inflict pain, discomfort and distance him from the loving care of his family. However, it is always challenging to help families see this. Knowing his interests and background, I put Pravin in charge of seeing this patient and discussing his care. To my surprise, he communicated empathetically with the patient's family and successfully brought them to the understanding that symptom management was more beneficial and dignified then invasive life support. Of course, it also helped that Pravin had met the family in home visits as a medical student and had already built a rapport with them.

As a medical student, Pravin has been involved in volunteer events for Star PALS, and various community operations/projects for children. After all that searching, he finally found home in paediatric palliative care. Pravin has a unique passion for really getting to know his patients, getting to know their struggles and even facing the struggles with them sometimes. He shares the joys and struggles of children (and their families) with chronic illnesses whose innocent childhood seems stolen and replaced by repeated medical battles. It stirs him to see the raw emotions brought about by simple everyday events taken for granted by others and this is beautifully reflected in his poems. *Storm Clouds* and *Take It Or Leave It* are daily contemplations, while *Wasted Time, To Live, To Breathe And To Feel*, and *Tell Me Where Your Heart Lies* are agonizing reflections of bereaved ones.

In *Fire, Faith and Glory*, the emotionally charged anthology of poems is inspired by our patients' lives and deaths. If you haven't seen what we've seen, then it is my hope the poems will give you an impression of a day in a life in the intensive care unit. If you have been in the unit as a family member or provider, the poems will help put words to the complex feelings you may have experienced and provide support in knowing that you are not alone. God bless.

Dr Judith Wong Ju-Ming,
Consultant,
Paediatric Intensive Care Unit,
KK Women's & Children's Hospital,
Singapore

# LETTER TO READERS

Fire, Faith & Glory commemorates my second year in Paediatric residency in KK Women's & Children's Hospital. It is an anthology of poems that brings you the readers through an emotional trajectory through my various postings across neonatology, high dependency and the children's intensive care unit. A sequel to *Do They Have Telephones Up in Heaven?*, this collection pays tribute to the children whom we have lost, children who have recovered well and children who are still fighting for their lives. This collection also remembers parents and their daily struggles through difficult times. I hope you will all find a poem in here that brings you comfort and heals any open wounds from past experiences. We all have a story to share and I am thankful to all the patients and their families who have inspired me to write these poems, each with their own little histories. As the title suggests, this anthology is fiercer, more intense and features poems which will make one reflect, persevere and strive towards a better tomorrow, which we are all working together for. I hope you will remember, as I always do, that you only get a beautiful rainbow after a heavy rain storm. And no matter how heavy, it will come to an end one day and the sun will shine again – brighter than ever before.

Peace, R R Pravin

# WASTED TIME

How will I ever
Undo wasted time
That one Sunday
I promised to
Bring you out
To the park

But I couldn't bring myself to
Cause I was too tired working
To pay off all your hospital bills
Sitting in my room waiting
Just like you were by my side
For an answer I didn't have

I can still remember
The sadness in your eyes
When I said I'm sorry son
Daddy has to work today

I can still remember
You walking away
Hiding your tears
Quietly sitting down
By yourself playing
With the old car
Your mum bought for you
When she was still around

1

Then the phone call came
One Sunday morning
Your Sunday school teacher
Said you'd met with an accident
The paramedics said they tried
But enough was not enough
For a grieving father
Who'd lost more than a child

I sat on the park bench
Your favourite one
And I reached out
But you weren't there
All I felt was an empty silence
That kept me company
And all I had left were regrets
Of wasted time I could have spent
Loving you more during your time
In this world.

**#Inspiration:**

"Wasted Time" is a poem I wrote after reading about how a child lost her life in a road accident. It showed that life was short and no one could predict when life could come to an abrupt end when one least expects it. This poem is written from a father's perspective for a child he lost. Time spent with our loved ones is timeless and priceless. There can be no value placed on it. It is important to cherish the little time we have with one another because when we lose a loved one, the regret, the guilt often accompany the sadness. This is also a special poem to me because I wrote it on my 25th birthday (23rd Oct '17) and it will always have that special significance. It is also a little something for bereaved families.

# FOR GOD'S CHILDREN IN
# HEAVEN & ON EARTH

I looked up today
Closing my eyes
In silent prayer
Hoping you'll
Remember the words
I said when you left

Darling I love you
I'm sorry for all
The pain and suffering
You had to endure
While you were
Alive on this Earth

In this lifetime
I hope no child
Has to suffer
As much as
You did

God please promise
Me you will heal
The children who
Are suffering,
Are crying for a cure
That no human love
Can ever provide for

There are days
When I look around
And wonder if
A child born to suffer
Would ever live a day
Without the pain
Without the worry
Of making it through another

For all the children
In heaven & on Earth
A little prayer
Can make a mile of a difference
To light a candle of hope
In the heart of a child
Broken by an anguish
None can comprehend

God I hope you hear
This quiet prayer
For a child to come
Or a child just passed,
That they shall always
Live a life filled with
Happiness only a child
Deserves to experience
On Earth & in heaven.

#Inspiration:

To all the angels in heaven & on Earth – I know the pain you went through or are going through. When I see the families in neonatal intensive care or in the children's cardiac step down unit, it is tough for them to watch their children go through major surgeries and stormy journeys, but I hope somewhere deep within, amidst the pain and suffering, they will know that their prayers will be heard. Sometimes, the answers aren't always straightforward but keeping the candle of hope makes a difference, how small or big.

# HOW ?

How can a life
So beautifully created
Be taken in an instant
Cremated to dust
Before its worth could be realised.

How can a wonder
That took nine months
To come to creation
Be gone in a moment
That can never come back.

How does a miracle
So skilfully moulded
Disappear and fade away
Before our very eyes
To a place only God has been.

How will I ever answer
My remaining children
Who will ask
Where big brother or sister have been
Though I know the answer
But just can't bear to say the words

How will I go on
Now that I'm alone
How do you expect me
To go on when part of me
Died with you

I ask myself
How will I ever heal?
How will I go on?
The answer I found
Lay right there with you
I have to go on
Because of you, for you
To carry on your legacy,
Your story, our struggles
So the world will know
That every life,
No matter how big or small,
Is precious

And each life
Is meant to be cherished
For you will never know
A life's full worth
Till the day it is truly gone.

I miss you. (we all do.)

**#Inspiration:**

How? was written because it is a question many parents and families ask when a tragedy such as the loss of a child hits them. The main question is 'How do we move on from here?' and it is a difficult one because it takes time, it takes great effort with a whole lot of emotion, to have the strength to pull through and carry on. But the main message is to remember that it is important to carry on the legacy and the story which somehow keeps the loved ones we've lost alive. It also is part of the gradual 'healing-from-the-hurt' process which takes time.

# GLORY

In my son's final hours
God give me the strength
To stand by his side
The very mother
Who can't bear to
Watch her own son
Die slowly before her eyes

Is this what life promised -
Hardship, ache and suffering
Every minute of every day
Of a child who did no wrong
To nobody in this world

Where is the justice
Lord I had so much faith
That you would make
My son's life better someday
Now here you make me
Stand witness to him
Ebbing away from our world
To join yours

All my life I praised your Name
And prayed with a faith
So unquestionable
No war can tear apart
Restore the glory in your Name
If you say you are truly the
Keeper of our children

Then save my child
When he joins you
Even though right now
It may seem as if
He is beyond saving
On this Earth
Please I beg of you

My child is my glory
My child is my life
My child is my breath
Take my heartbeat away
And all I am left with
Is an empty body
Without a beating heart

God grant my child
A divine dignity
Only you have the power to restore
Please give my child back his glory,
The glory of being a child, my son.

# #Inspiration:

I wrote this poem during my second year in residency when I had a young child who was had end stage kidney failure and was not a candidate for dialysis or kidney transplant. I was asked to be with them when the child acutely deteriorated and I was with the parents through their most trying moments – which was coming to terms with accepting that this may be the last time they would be seeing their child. The part that made me tear and write this poem was when they called a priest to the room to say a prayer and the priest himself broke down during the prayer. And that moved me to tears which I had to fight back because the parents were already devastated and a part of me knew I had to remain strong for the child and the family.

# FIRE

A fire burns
Within my womb
My child is dying
The doctors say
Ending my world
In just four words

The raging tears
Are too hard
To hold back
Ravaging my once
Perfect world with
My beautiful kid

Someone spread
The word to pray
Harder for a child
Who is leaving
This world too soon

The inferno of love
Burns within my veins
A love so fierce
That a part of me
Wants my child
To feel the power of
A mother's love
And fight to come back

Set fire to the
Non-believers
There is a flicker of hope
That remains in this woman
I will not give up so easily
This mother is not going
Down without a fight
A quiet petition of faith
To bring my child back to me

They say my child
May be dying
But here she lies breathing
Every moment counts
To the end,
Any kid's final battle
Will ignite a flame so powerful
In a mother wanting to protect
Her child from the claws of death

Once a spark starts,
It will spread like wildfire
Like it has within this mother.


#Inspiration:

It is a natural instinct for mothers to protect their children. When a child is dying, a mother will do all she can to stop death from taking her child. It will light a fire that is beyond control. This poem aims to capture just that because there is no fire that burns brighter than a fire that burns within a woman for her dying child.

# STORM CLOUDS

Sometimes storm clouds
Hover above us
Blocking out the sunshine
Filling our days
With a darkness too deep
And too painful to bear

These clouds come
And these clouds go
But the puddles
They leave behind
May forever
Mar our souls

Remember to stand tall
With your umbrella
And never bend
To the sorrows
Of a storm
That shall one day pass

Though it may seem
That life's impossible
To live when rainy days
Rain harder than hail
Hold on tight to your raincoat
And never yield to the storm clouds

I believe
One day
Storm clouds will go
And the sun will shine once more.

**#Inspiration:**

Everyone has their rainy days but I hope this poem will bring a little light and a little encouragement for those who feel like it has been so hard all these years. Living with a child or a loved one with a complex illness can be difficult and even being that person having to live and struggle through a complex illness is unthinkable. But please do believe that the rain will stop and the sun will shine again someday. Much love.

# LAST WISH

I will always remember
How Charlie never got
His last wish

He was a little kid
Who loved to go to church
And hear the others sing
And he would rejoice with them
Never really understanding
What was going on
But he knew somehow
That Sunday mornings
Were always a good time
To hear a person called
God share his word

Charlie wasn't like
All the other kids
He was born a little shorter
He didn't look like the rest
But that did not matter
Cause Mummy always said
He was special
And so did *Mickey*,
His favourite mouse on Earth

One day he came to the hospital
And he felt something was not right
This admission wasn't like the previous
He felt that he was going to miss
His Mummy and *Mickey*
And he may never be able
To go to church that Sunday

We did all we could
To make his wish come true
But before Sunday came
Charlie couldn't breathe too well
His mum teared knowing
That Charlie's last wish
May not come true.

**#Inspiration:**

When I was finishing my paediatric high dependency posting as a second year resident, I met a lovely child and his family. Their final wish for him before he passed due to progression of his chronic illness was for him to attend a special church event. We had prepared everything the week prior and there was some hope that he would be able to make it. However, just a day or two before, he deteriorated and we had to cancel all the special arrangements we made just so that his last wish could be fulfilled. It was heart-wrenching for all of us and I just couldn't imagine how the child would have felt. These are difficult moments that are unpredictable and it makes us appreciate how important last wishes are to everyone.

# TO LIVE, TO BREATHE & TO FEEL

Isn't life a beautiful thing
To live, to breathe and to feel
Each and every morning

But then a child
In a world far away
Lays silently still
In a hospital room
On life support
And a breathing machine
Waiting for a chance
To live life again

Sadly the chance never comes
And the child never gets
To live, to breathe and to feel
Life again like he once used to

Like how he always celebrated a birthday
Or like how he always made his mother laugh
When he accidentally spilt milk all over
Her brand new dress one evening
And she got so angry that she stopped
And started laughing because
She knew every moment with him
Was a precious one that will someday matter

Like how he once made his nephrologist
Feel how fortunate she was to have a patient
Who made her day every time he came to clinic
With a smile so special that it'll melt her heart
Till she too shed a tear the day she knew
There'll be an empty vacancy in her clinic
During the 4 o'clock slot he was always scheduled for

He made the nurses in the ward
Remember how lucky they were
To live, to breathe and to feel
For the children they cared for
At home and in the hospital
For every child's life was one
Not to be taken for granted

Isn't life a beautiful thing
One day we have it in our hands
And the next day it slips away
Won't you stop and take a moment
To remember
To live,
To breathe and
To always feel the life around
And the life within.

**#Inspiration:**

I wrote this poem as a dedication to a patient we lost recently in the ward I was posted to. Though we knew his time would be up soon, it is always sad to hear of a child's passing. On one hand, it teaches all of us to appreciate life a little more. On the other, my heart goes out to the parents who raised a child for a good number of years. There is an unspoken rule that the older the child gets, the harder it is to lose them. I was scrolling through the list of patients and when I realised the name of the patient I helped to look after was gone, a part of me hoped that he had a terminal discharge and went home to pass on in peace. Sadly, he passed on in the ward after a party he had – I guess he held on for as long as he could. Life is an enigma – I have honestly not figured it out yet but I hope it will be kind to children who deserve to live long special lives. And always take a moment to live, to breathe and to always feel the life & love around. Peace xx.

# TELL ME WHERE YOUR HEART LIES

Dearest child
Tell me where your heart lies
Is it on this Earth
Or in the world yonder

Your time with us
Was far too short
Your sudden leaving
Broke us into pieces

Maybe there were times
When we weren't the
Best parents you wanted
But please don't go

So many things
Life planned for us
Just as we had waited
A long time for you

Now that you may
Already be gone
Just a body
With a departed soul

Far and beyond
Into another world
Where your heart
Lies free and happy

Cause if you have
Already left us
I hope you'll know
We will always love you
Our precious one & only,
We miss you.

**#Inspiration:**

During my children's intensive care rotation, I met a child who had suffered brain damage after choking on food. The child's parents were devastated and were in shock. They had waited for a long time to have this child and to have their child suddenly taken from them was unfortunately extremely tragic. Part of them had hope that their child will return and they called priests from various religious denominations to come and to pray. My heart went out to them and to their child. Though I knew the child was physically there in the intensive care, I knew the child's heart was in another world beyond – free from this one. This experience also made me understand that a parent's love for their child is one that is beyond measure.

# LETTING GO

Have we been
Holding on
For far too long
Or are we just being
Parents who love
Their child too much

Everyone tells us
It is time to let go
But no one knows
What it means
Having to pull the plug
On your child

The guilt, the pain
The regret, the sleepless nights
Revisiting the painful memories
Of the ambulance ride
Of the demoralising family meetings
Of the endless 'I'm sorry for your loss'

Just when we thought
We had finally become
One happy family
You decide to leave us
Leaving us barren

Why didn't we love you
More than we could
When you were still around
Now that it's too late
To say 'Son I love you'

We know you left us
After we started the CPR*
A little too late
No amount of medication
Or prayer can bring you back
(Trust us we have tried)

I can't imagine
I am writing this
Maybe it is time
To say goodbye after all.

**#Inspiration:**

For parents to let go of their child in an acute setting such as the children's intensive care unit is extremely difficult. Often, it is a sudden sentinel event that no one is prepared for. Early involvement of the symptom care team is important to help build a rapport with and support the distraught parents through trying times. No parent ever wants to let go. As humans, it will make them feel as if they did not do everything they could for their child and in their distraught states, they will not be able to take a step back and be objective like the medical team often is. It is never easy and it is the worst nightmare ever for a parent. Goodbye remains the hardest word ever to be said, all the more to a child.

*CPR stands for Cardiopulmonary Resuscitation*

# PLEASE NO MORE

There comes a point
When I stopped calling
The doctors monsters
The nurses devils
Who tried to take my child

I knew none of it
Was going to change
The course of my child's illness
It was moving faster than
Any of us could keep up with

I used to be angry,
Mad, sad, upset
But right now
I know there is no point
In any of that anymore
Cause it won't save my child

All the hours I spent
Running between
Home and hospital
Looking after my
Other children
All alone as a single parent
Will have all been in vain

All the time
I thought you'd come home
Back to mummy, the baby
Everyone called a miracle
Cause you came out so early
Yet you survived like a hero
You've always been to Mummy

What will I tell your older sister
Who's waiting for you to come home
That maybe it was all a dream
My dream I made so many mistakes in
Time and medications can never reverse

How much more
Must this Mother suffer
God please no more
There is only so much
A human heart can take.

#### #Inspiration:

Sitting in a family conference for a child on ECMO (extracorporeal membrane oxygenation support which is often used for children who are extremely unwell as an artificial heart-lung support), I remember a mother who was really upset with the entire healthcare system. But during this particular family conference, the news that her child may never make it, was broken to her. For the first time, this mother who always had a brave demeanour, broke down and said 'I knew it'. She then said 'All my anger is not going to save my child. Nothing is going to save my child'. My heart sank when she broke into inconsolable tears. It was the hardest thing for a single mother to hear and she also added 'No other baby should ever have to go through this.'

# NO OTHER

No other child
Should have to suffer
The way you did
Ever since you were born

There is so much
A body can bear
And you've been
Through more
Than any can imagine

First the tubes
Now a heart-lung machine
And all these injections
Sometimes I feel
I don't recognise
The happy child I once knew

All these battle scars
Hopefully will pay off
Someday – when you'll
Live to tell your story
Just as I will mine

I'm sorry if this life
Hasn't been a piece of cake
But I hope it will get better
Mummy promises it will.

**#Inspiration:**

Often when infants and children are admitted to the neonatal intensive care unit or the children's intensive care unit, parents are very much affected when they see their children intubated with multiple lines in-situ. However, remaining hopeful is crucial and parents often ask what they can do within their capacity to help their child. Often, the answer is to be there and talk to their children because they can hear, they can feel and they somehow know – that is a magical thing I will never be able to explain but it is the magic and mystery of the human touch, a powerful bond between parent and child.

# DEAR BELOVED

Dear sweet child of mine
Can you ever tell me why
You chose to come to
A world that may not have been
Too ready to accept you angel

Your time with us
Was as quick as lightning
That I find myself
Trying to remember
The day you came
And how soon after
You left me

Dear beloved angel
Tell me is this what
Destiny wanted for us
To meet for a moment
Only to never see each other
For an eternity more

I wish time was a little
More generous to me
So that I could hold you
A moment longer
Without having to beg
Or bargain with the angels
Who had come to take you
To another world
Far away from me

Dear beloved child
I hope God will be kind
Enough to give me
A second chance
To be a parent
To another child
Like you.

#Inspiration:

Dear Beloved is a simple poem I penned one Sunday morning after watching a video commemorating children who had passed over a year at « Le Phare » (The Lighthouse), a non-profit organisation in Montréal that looks after children with paediatric palliative care needs and helps their families. It was a really lovely video that captured the happiest moments for each of the children who had passed and soon after this poem was born in honour of their little legacies.

# CAN YOU HEAR

Can you hear
The summer rains calling
Your name looking for
A child they lost
A monsoon ago

Can you hear
The angels singing
Your name in praise
Of a child they found
One Christmas ago

Can you hear
Your father remembering
Your name to hold on
To memories that sometimes
Seem so far away

Can you hear
Your mother crying
Your name each year
When it is time
To light a candle
On your altar

Can you hear
Your little brother pronouncing
Your name bit by bit
Learning the alphabet and
Learning about his older sister

Can you hear
The doctors and nurses saying
Your name at mortality meetings
Trying to immortalise another patient
They lost all too suddenly

Can you hear
The winter winds singing
Your name as they lay a
Magic wreath where you rest
Hoping you'd remember
That we've not forgotten.


**#Inspiration:**

I have always wondered when children leave us, if they do look down from above and listen to us reminiscing about them – be it their parents, their family or even the hospital staff who once looked after them. I've always believed that those who left us somehow can still hear us as I believe my Dad can sometimes hear what I'm thinking or saying. Maybe and hopefully it is the same with all the children cause it will be our way of keeping them alive in our hearts.

# MARCH TO THE FINISH

Son, you've put on
Such a brave fight
All your life

All this time
Without a stir
Without a flinch
You ploughed
Through the hard times

We will finish
This race together
March on to the end
And no one can
Try to stop us now

Father and son
Man to man
We will make it

**#Inspiration:**

Often when times get rough, a parent's courage and faith in their child somehow inspires a fighting spirit in the child. There is no scientific explanation for this but heart to heart, it makes a quiet huge difference. This poem is a battle cry from a father to his ill son who is turning the corner, representing a beacon of hope and light.

# WAR MEMORIAL

When your time is up
I'll sound the horns
May all the warriors
Who fought before
Await your arrival
And welcome you
With open arms

The guns will fire
And the bagpipes will play
We will march along
Your glorious casket
Telling your story
In a eulogy so powerful
The world will remember
Your legacy

You were only five
But you fought wars
No soldier has before
You were a hero
To the children around
You are now a veteran,
A martyr

You came home to us
Wrapped in your favourite blanket,
The flag that wrapped your coffin
And will follow you through
To the world after where
There shall be no more wars
For innocent children

We march on forth
In your loving memory.

**#Inspiration:**

Whenever a child dies, it feels like we lost a soldier in the war against an illness be it cancer or otherwise. Every child that passes fighting a war so heavy against maladies deserves a send-off equivalent to or greater than a war hero because these children are martyrs. They are special martyrs who will live on in all our hearts and in all our memories.

# TAKE IT OR LEAVE IT

God stop playing
These childish games
With us parents

You either take our child
Or you leave our child with us
Please don't keep us hanging on

Somedays you make us feel
Recovery is well on its way
And on others there is no hope

Life is not an in-between
There is no grey
Only black or white

We never did wrong
Please don't make
Our dear daughter suffer

A child is a child
An innocently pure life
That deserves nurturing
And not suffering

So take it or leave it God
Don't leave us helplessly
Holding on to empty hope

Whatever the outcome
We will be ready
Or at least try to be.

**#Inspiration:**

It is tough for parents especially when sometimes they feel that their child is getting better and on other days, the outcome remains bleak. There is no clear or straightforward answer that the medical team can provide, leaving the parents hanging on. Sometimes these are honest questions that parents will have on their minds. And hanging on helplessly in-between, neither here nor there, is unimaginably tough. This poem represents an honest conversation a parent has with God to answer a bigger question no one human can.

# REFLECTIONS

Everyone wants to save a child
What if the child comes too late
And we can't turn back the clock

It's terrible when we can't save
Cause that's what we were built to do
And we reflect, wondering what can be done
Better the next time, although
Hopefully there won't be a similar next time

Parents scream, relatives yell
Blaming the medical team for
A loss nothing can compensate for
But we tried too, we never gave up

We all have children we wished
That reached the hospital earlier
But sometimes we are limited
For we are not Gods
And no - we can't play God.

**#Inspiration:**

This is a poem written from the perspective of a medical personnel. While doctors and nurses do their best to save every child, it is a rough reality when there are prolonged downtimes resulting in the child not reaching the hospital early enough with a sad ending. There is no one to be blamed and it is inevitable. But that doesn't keep us from trying our best to save every child's life cause every life matters – to all of us.

# THE OTHER WAY ROUND

As I lay down
These memories of old
I think of you
And your smile
That melted
A thousand hearts
Mine being first in line.

I really loved you
The way a parent
Should love a child –
Unconditionally.

I wish I could
Have made all
Your dreams
Come true –

But how can
A broken heart
Bleeding for
His son's return
Ever make
Forgotten dreams
A reality again.

There are days
When I close my eyes
And imagine you
Standing here
Right next to me,
Your tiny hand in mine
And your little shoelace undone
Waiting for Big Daddy to bend down
And tie that little knot for you.

Your passing
Took my only
Meaningful job away
That was to serve you
Day and night
And to love you
Like no other.

Here I stand
Facing the epitaph
I wrote for you –
'Here lies the Greatest
Son who ever lived'
Wishing it had been
The other way round
With you standing here
Remembering me instead.

**#Inspiration:**

Whenever a child passes, parents always ask 'Why couldn't it have been me instead?' and this poem hopes to capture just that. Often children read eulogies for their parents but when a child passes, it is the other way round. It is an odd feeling parents have, many a time wishing it could have been them instead. It is a natural reaction and it is sad because children are meant to live on but not all of them have a chance to.

# SECOND OPINION

Sometimes I wish
For a piece of good news
From someone else

I can deal no more
With the pain
The sadness
That comes with hearing –

It's over.
Cause if it's over
How will we make it
Through each long day
Without caressing you
In our tender, loving arms

Somedays we walk away
In the other direction
When the doctors come
Cause we know all they bring
Is a reality that we will never
Ever be able to face,
A reality without our child

We've asked everywhere
Out of a desperation so deep
Hoping that someone somewhere
Will give us something we want to hear

Please hear us out
Our minds know the truth
But it is one too heavy for
Our feeble hearts to bear.


**#Inspiration:**

Accepting a child's sudden death in the children's intensive care unit setting is difficult for any parent and often they seek second opinions from either a traditional doctor or from a specialist from another hospital who often shares the same grim news with them. However, as parents it is their way of expressing that they have done everything they could before they agree to withdrawal of care. It is a difficult call to make as we will never understand the immense grief and suffering the parents are going through during such a difficult time.

# DEAR TEDDY

Dear Teddy,
Glad to have you
Right here beside me
As I lay fast asleep
In eternal sleep

While I watch above
On a cloud in heaven
I see my family crying
Asking me to return
Promising me a trip to Disneyland
That is never going to happen –
Not in this lifetime at least

I see the doctors and nurses
Walking past in a sad silence
Trying to keep me comfortable
Pulling a blanket over me
And making sure you are nestled
Comfortably next to me

Thank you
For keeping me company
When all life had left me
The moment I collapsed
Remaining faithfully by
My side in quiet peace.

Funny how people cry
Once we have left
Teddy I wish they'd
Remember my smile
And the happy times
We shared as a family

Dear Teddy,
Now that I'm gone
Hope you'll follow me
To the new world after,
You're my one and only
Best toy buddy forever.


**#Inspiration:**

When I examined a child who was brain dead, I always made sure he had
his teddy bear snuggled next to him. It may be surprising to us but such
little toys have huge significance in the lives of these children even though
they may not be alive anymore by medical definition. It offers a comfort to
them and their families because it is a peaceful image of not a child dying
but rather a child in eternal sleep.

# WHEN I DIE

When I leave this world
I want to leave a hero
I want all the leaders
To sing praises of a
Special child who
Loved to live life
To the fullest

When I die
I hope I will
Meet angels
Who will play with me
In a playground filled with
Children who passed before me
Where we can be happy in unity

When I die
I wish for
Everyone to be happy
And not be sad
Because you all made me
So happy when I was alive

When I am no longer with you
I hope you will continue to love
Other children after me
As you loved me
Maybe a new brother or sister
Whom I may never meet
But tell them I love them

After I die
I hope I would have
Changed this world
To make it a better place
For all children to live
Happily ever after

**#Inspiration:**

I wrote this poem after imagining a child writing a poem dedicated to all the children in the world. This is a special poem because a child only wishes for the best for everyone – his family and his friends. This child's poem will also help parents find peace in a child's departure because there is yet a renewed hope in the future. The closing of one chapter does not mean the end but rather it paves the way for a new beginning – a new happily ever after.

# LITTLE COFFIN

It is hard to see
A little coffin
One that holds
A heart so little

A little coffin
That deserves
A big send off

A little coffin
That I'll miss

Rest in peace.

**#Inspiration:**

It is difficult for anyone to see a little coffin, because it means that a little heart is now gone forever on this Earth. Each stanza is a line shorter than the previous because sometimes we are simply at a loss for words. Rest in peace little ones – we miss you.

# THE HAPPY POEM

Look around
And you will see
The colours of
A world of beauty

In each child's eyes
A hope blooms
A rainbow shines
Through life's storms

Hardship precedes
A life of happiness
There can be no
Poem without pain
And no song
Without sorrow

Search within
The sad times
And you will find
A strength
Like no other

When you feel
Like giving up
Cause the storm clouds
Don't seem to be clearing up
Look up to the blue sky
And remember you story
Is being written day by day
With a beautiful ending
Waiting for you at the very end
Where your dreams come true
And you find your happiness
Ever after.

**#Inspiration:**

For all parents, siblings and anyone going through a difficult time, this poem is for you. There are days when nothing seems to be working out fine but remember that this is part of life's journey. Sometimes it takes a while for you to find the answer but we will eventually get there. Once we do, we will look back and be grateful we safely reached the other end of the rainbow where only happiness awaits us.

# REMEMBER ME

Remember me
By the love I
Always spread
To make you smile

Remember me
By the hugs I
Used to give
To make your day better

Remember me
By the songs I
Always sang
To cheer you up

Remember that
When you bury me
Bury my body but
Don't bury my words

Don't take this life
For granted because
Everyone is given
Only one life
Once you lose it,
There is no retrieving it

Live it like
It is all that you have
And that you will never
Have another
To say I love you
To the ones you cherish


**#Inspiration:**

Written from the persona of a little child, this poem serves as a reminder
to all parents to remember their children for all the lovely moments they
shared together. A child's words also carry much wisdom. It is important
to immortalise these words which would forever live in our hearts.

# TINY DANCER

Every day I see
Children come
And children go
I am all that remains
In a ward that seems to
Grow old with me

I look at the window
And see children
Being carried home
By happy parents
Unlike mine
Who seem worried
All the time

I used to dance
When I was young
But now with all
These drips and treatments
Hooked onto me
My freedom is gone

All I have
Is a music box
Where a tiny ballerina
Dances in a little circle
To comfort me
When I feel a tear
Or two coming on

How I wish
I could be that tiny dancer
That goes round and round
In circles in a perfect world
Where time comes to a standstill
With only happy melodies and
No sadness or suffering at all

I wish I could
Go back in time
And tell myself
This life will be tough
Tiny dancer,
Don't you ever lose
That little rhythm
That beats strong
In your little heart

**#Inspiration:**

I wrote this poem with a little child in mind watching a tiny ballerina
dancing on a music box. The power of a music box has a lot of significance
in my life because when I am sad, I do turn on the little music box I
have. Though it only plays Christmas songs, it somehow cheers me up.
In this poem, a child remembers how she was a little dancer once upon a
time when she looks at her music box, which for her serves as a symbol of
strength and courage.

# REASON

Young one,
I know what you are
Going through seems
Tougher than you can imagine
But listen,
Your dreams are waiting
To be told
Your hopes are waiting
To be realised
Your story is one
That will live on forever

Olympians have won
Gold medals they were
Forever remembered for,
When you pull through
Life will award you a
Golden star that will
Inspire other children
To be just like you

Your time is not up yet
There are so many more
Moments for you to live,
The pain may take away
What will there is to live
But hold on won't you
To see another sunrise

Mummy and Daddy
Never gave up on you
Then why must you
Even think of letting go

Yes I know
There are days
When you wished
You never woke up
But child listen
We were all meant
To live for a reason
Though you may not see it now
Someday you will understand
Your purpose and your reason.

**#Inspiration:**

This poem hopes to give everyone who wants to give up, a reason to live again. Though we may not understand our purpose now, someday the reason will be clear and we will look back at our lives not with regret but with a smile of gratitude that we knew our purpose, our reason.

# JOSEPH'S DREAM

I have a dream
That all children
Will never get cancer
And have to suffer
Like me

I have a dream
That all children
Will never need
Ports or ever need
To be poked with needles
Those sharp and scary monsters

I have a dream
That all children
Will live in big, bouncy castles
With an endless supply of candy
And wishes from magical fairies

I have a dream
That all children
Will never know
The meaning of pain
Or medications
Wish I never knew
What chemotherapy meant
The poison that made me
Lose all my brown hair

I have a dream
That all children
Will never have to say
Goodbye to their parents
Like I had to before
They gave me morphine
Again another poison
To kill the pain
That took my childhood away

I have a dream
That all children
Reading this
Will be selfless like me
And continue to wish
The best for all children
Like me and you

**#Inspiration:**

This poem is written from a child's perspective. Children with oncological conditions often suffer through the trauma of chemotherapy, port accessing with needles and endure pain beyond belief. In this poem, Joseph wishes the best for all the children in generations ahead of him in a premature obituary he writes in the form of this poem.

# WHAT WAS (NEVER) MEANT TO BE

Though I'll never
Know your name
And never had
A chance to hold you
In my arms
I hope you'll forgive me

When they scanned me
I was so excited to see you
But then something was wrong
The cardiologist looked at me
And said this may not last
And my heart broke in two
One for me, and one for you

The geneticist was next
All the specialties a blur
All I remember was them saying
You had to go, cause even after
You were born, you'd leave soon after
Cause you weren't meant to stay

My world fell apart
It was me and you
Against the world
I then realised
It wouldn't be fair for you
To live a life of unhappiness
And you'd look at me
Wondering why I made the choice I made
Only to punish you in this cruel world

The day came when I said
My final goodbye to you
You whom I'll never know
I hope you'll thank me someday
For all the suffering I saved you from
Though it didn't save me from
My own guilt and sadness

Sometimes I guess
What was meant to be
Will be, though a little part of me
Always wished I'd known you better.


**#Inspiration:**

During my paediatric genetics and cardiology postings, there were mothers
I knew of who underwent termination of pregnancies after much discussion
with each of the specialists due to the non-viability of the foetus. Though
it may seem a simple matter, it leaves a huge impact on these mothers
who are often emotional in clinic and endure a lot of suffering in silence.
It is important to offer them antenatal palliative care in the form of
bereavement and to follow up accordingly. One can only imagine what a
mother goes through including the emotional rollercoaster of events. It is
not an easy decision and it is never a piece of news an expectant mother
wants to hear. Hence it is important to support these mothers through
these difficult times.

# GOD BLESS THE RAINS (OF MIRACLES)

Tears of joy shed
For a child who broke the
Spell of illness and who lives

Dancing in celebration
With a child who reigns
Supreme in fiery remission
From a cancer everyone
Once thought was undefeatable

Singing in praise
Of a child who walked again
After an accident that could have
Left the weak at heart crippled

God bless the rains
Of miracles that are
Falling upon all of
Our children

Word spread across
The street like a wildfire
Of miracles of children
Magically recovering from
Mysterious maladies of old

Cheer on the children
Who believed in themselves
More than ever to heal again

Come hurry on parents
See for yourselves
That anything is possible
In a world of faith and hope

God bless the rains
Of miracles that are
Falling upon all of
Our children
Here on now, today
And forever more!

**#Inspiration:**

An uplifting anthem for all the children that have come out of the darkness of their illness – this one is for you and your families! God bless you and your families – and for those going through a rough patch, don't give up – it will be your turn soon to receive the rains of blessings filled with miracles from up above!

# HOLD YOU (TILL FOREVER)

I will hold you
Till forever
And never let you go
Little son of mine

I once held a daughter
Whom I lost too soon
And I won't let that
Ever happen to me again

I may be a young father
Whom the elders frown upon
Me and my wife's bad luck
For having lost two children

What does it matter to the rest
When it is you losing your child
The words they say don't mean
Nothing because they only fade away

There is no way I am
Going to lose you
The doctors said
You were born blue
But to me your smile
Is as pink as can be

I know it is selfish of me
To ask of you to stay with me
And to never leave me
To join your sister who like
You left all too soon
When she was born blue

Come back to Papa
Won't you so I know
That you love me
As much as I love you.


**#Inspiration:**

During my cardiology posting, there were neonatal cases of babies born with cyanotic heart disease who did not make it despite extensive resuscitation due to poor oxygenation from the underlying cardiac condition. While I was preparing a medical summary for one of such patients, this poem came to mind and I immediately penned it down as a tribute to all the 'blue' babies who have since passed on. You are not forgotten and will never be.

# SEPTEMBER FLOWERS

September flowers
For the child who
Made it through
All the months
And all the mountains
Of hurt and pain

Every day
A new milestone
A new congratulations
For the brave kid
Who fought his demons
And is winning

Keep going
October is just
Round the corner
And by then
Hopefully
You will be cured.


**#Inspiration:**

I wrote this poem after having a moment's imagery of flowers and this little piece of courage came soon after I had initially planned to complete the compilation actually. Hope you like it! Keep fighting young ones – the world is waiting and has much in store for you! xx

# CANCEL THE CANCER

Cancer you know
I'm not a fool
You can't trick me
Into thinking
I can't beat you!

I always dreamt
I could be anything
And you won't ever
Take that away
From me, no you won't!

I used to see the
World in colour
Till you ruined it
Making it
Only black and white
But no one is ever
Going to take
The rainbow out of me!

You may have
Taken others before me
But I will show you
That together
The human spirit
Is invincible!

People say
Cry out the cancer
I'm done crying
Time for me
To stand up to you
Like a pretty victim
To a baseless bully
Start praying
Cause I'm so done
With you!

Time to cancel out
The cancer and
Live life as it is!

**#Inspiration:**

Cancel the Cancer was pretty much a poem written from a teenager's point of view when truth be told, they express their sentiments with honesty and it comes to a point when they are done arguing with cancer and simply want to move on with the conversation of their lives – which is exactly what I hope to capture here.

# P.K.U (PRETTY, KOOL, UNIQUE)

I may look
Just a bit different
From you, from him, from her
But that don't matter

Genetics made me
But your words
Don't hurt me,
Accept me
For all my antics
Cause there is
Only ever gonna be
One copy of me

Special therapies
I'll always be on
Keeping me alive
Moving on and on

Sometimes it's expensive
But life don't have a price
Cause I was born this way
Treatment is not child's play

Some have the answers
Others never find one
Cause syndromes are a mystery
I can't even pronounce mine
But we still make history
With genes so unique
We live everyday cool and unfazed
By the funny looks and stares
We get from people who look
As strange to us

I may be different
But you can bet
I'm just as
P.K.U
As you!

**#Inspiration:**

This was really a fun record of sorts written from a perspective of a child who may look uniquely differently cool from others due to an underlying genetic condition. I wrote it during my genetics posting when I saw one of the three patients with PKU (phenylketonuria) which is a condition where there is a decreased breakdown of a particular protein subunit in the body in clinic. The title is derived from the condition of the same name and this fun poem was born! (it also has little rap undertones to it so for any child feeling the heat of being different, just rap this out to your friends and you will be reminded that not everyone can be as P.K.U (Pretty, *K*ool, Unique) as you!). Peace xx.

# LISTEN LITTLE ANGEL

Hospital to hospital
We ran this race
To bring you back
To the beautiful baby girl
You once were

Like a candle
You lit
A flicker of hope
In our hearts
Each time you smiled
We hoped
You were getting better

Then one day
Your heart gave way
The machines ran
To your aid
Breathing for you
And living for you

Every one tried
To bring you back to
The way you once were
But you decided
Your time here was up

That day plays over
And over again
In Mummy's mind
Your pain, my fears
All coming back
Hitting me hard
Sometimes that
You've moved on
Though you were
Still here with us

Goodbye my child
Time won't bring
Your heart back to us
I never dreamt
That I will live to
See the day
I lose you

Though you may
Have gone your own way
Please remember
Mummy and Daddy,
We will always walk with you
Till we see you again
One sweet day

Every time
I imagine heaven
And how far away and lonely
It must be for you
I hope you find family
And friends to love you
And play with you
And raise you like their own
I will thank them
When I join you someday

My tears are
Only for you
I love you
I'm sorry
I lost you,
I love you.

Listen little angel,
Heaven sent,
Mummy has to say
Goodbye for now
Your friends await.

**#Inspiration:**

Dedicated to a mum who decided to let go of her child, this one is for you and your child. We will miss you. You have put up a strong and brave fight. It is never easy to let go. I remember accompanying this child on a hospital to hospital transfer. When we said goodbye, we hoped that we will meet again with news that she was getting better. However, when I received news that the child suffered from brain injury after a long resuscitation and mum was letting go, it was sad to think of all that the mum and the child had gone through. I wrote this for them and my heart is with them all the way.

# THE ONE THING THAT
# MEANT THE MOST

Wish I had a
Little more time
To say
I miss you
Before I lost you

Old friends,
Old relatives
Ask why you left
All too young
I look at them
In silence

Not all questions
Have easy answers

I look at the
Empty house
And sometimes
I hear your voice
Calling me Papa

Then I turn around
And realise
You are no more

There are times
When I'd walk
For miles in the rain
Hoping to get rid
Of all this pain

Never planned
On dealing with
The death of my son
This early on in life

This life is full
Of surprises I can't explain
Tell me God
What you'd hoped to tell me
By hurting me this way
And taking away
The one thing that
Meant the most to
A once proud father

**#Inspiration:**

I wrote this poem in honour of all the fathers who have fought long and hard battles for their children. Being a father in the face of adversity especially when their child is in a critical condition is not easy – they have to play the dual role of supporting the family and not letting their guard down. But it is alright to shed a tear because sometimes that helps to relieve a lot of the stress, anxiety and pain. This is a tribute to all the fathers out there!

# TRAVELLING NORTH

I've walked a long
Time missing a leg
And missing on life

Mum I wanted you
To know that I
Did all I could to live

But it is time
For me to
Travel north

If you ever worry
Let me promise you
I'll be okay, maybe better

At least
I'll be beautiful again
With both feet
And maybe for once
I will feel
Whole again

**#Inspiration:**

This poem was penned from a perspective of a teenager with a bone tumour requiring an amputation talking to her parents in her final hours. It is already hard to lose part of oneself physically and sometimes the children lose more than that. My ultimate wish for these kids is to feel whole again when they enter a new world up north, up above.

# A PARENT'S PRAYER

I can see the light
And it's burning
Ever so brightly
Guess it's time
For me to go
I'll see you
Again someday

We've rode on
This wagon of life
Now the wheels
Have all worn out
Time for the rusty engine
To head home to retire

God I pray
You'll give me
The will
To move on
In peace

Don't look back
Don't hurry on
All we have is now
And that's all that
Really matters
Cause once I'm gone
All you'll have
Are memories
Of us now

Baby don't cry
Baby don't tear
You know
I'll always be here
Call me when
You need me
I'll still be here.


**#Inspiration:**

This poem was written when I recollected how hard it is for a child to lose their parent when they are young. This is for all you readers out there who lost a parent when you were young cause I know how it feels. No matter how far they may seem sometimes, the actual truth is they never left and will always be watching from up above. They would want us to move on in their name, their memory and their legacy.

# SHINE!

Surfing through my sickness
Riding on the waves
Of resilience
No one's gonna take
Away my shine

Life's not always
Pebbles and beaches
But not letting this
Get the best of me
My dreams will come true

Walking down
School hallways
Owning my stride
Though I may be bald
With tubes and scars
All over my body
Let me remind you
These are but accessories
To my special individuality

Will rise high above
The chains (and lines) that
Bind me to
Cancer blues

I will survive,
Shine bright and clear
For years to come
For nothing's ever
Gonna break
My shine!

**#Inspiration:**

This poem is dedicated to all the children fighting cancer or any chronic illness. Own your illness and own your shine! You're undefeatable as long as you believe in you.

# POWER REMIX

Have all these words in me
Wanna pen 'em down
From A to Z
Sometimes I feel
Nobody really can see
Who the real me is

I am but a
Nine-year-old
Behind this disease
They have yet
To really find a name for

I may seem
Smaller than
What I have
But who daresay
I can't defeat
This maladie

Try to drown me
With a diagnosis
Too much to bear

Come on let this
Little teddy bear
Break it down for you
Little me has a power
That's gon' make
Any sickness cower
Cause I will rise
And finally tower
High and above

Who said
Ain't nobody
Can remix
Fate & destiny
Just because
You see me
Enjoying my
Peanut, butter & jelly
Don't mean
I am too young to rally
All my power to
Send you back to
Where you came from

Bad genies don't deserve
To be free from their lamps
I am gonna unwish you
Ever existed
So no other child will have to
Suffer like me

Who says
Boys can't play with dolls
And girls can't play with cars
Likewise who says
Sick kids can't get better

Children of the world
Are you in this with me
We've got the pow-, pow-
POWER!


**#Inspiration:**

This is simply an all-time fun rap style poem that is highly contemporary
and you can imagine an army of babies or children dropping their pacifiers
and rocking out with dem shades and rattles! I hope you have as much fun
reading this as I did creating it – Peace Out!

# SIXTEEN HOURS

Sixteen hours
And sixteen minutes
Since you been gone
Into the operating theatre

I can't even eat
Thinking of all
The hours you
Were fasted
Your hunger
Burns within me

They told me
This could be
The final operation
For you to relieve
The pressures
Troubling your mind

I've had you
For sixteen years
And each time
I see you go
Through a new scan
To see that tumour,
I think of the day
You turned one

I remember
We celebrated
Your birthday
At a fancy restaurant
And I said
Cheers to sixty more

But here I am
Sitting alone
In the waiting room
Counting down
To the moment
I see you again
Cause I may lose you
Anytime now

Call me crazy
But I just want
The best for you
Till your last

Tell me
Doesn't a mother
Need her peace
Knowing she did
All she could
For her only son

**#Inspiration:**

I penned this little poem after I spent some time in the operating theatre during my anaesthesia elective. Little surgeries for children are scary for them and even scarier for their parents whom I see pacing in the waiting room. This took me back to a moment when a teenager with a metastatic brain tumour underwent a shunt insertion for symptom relief. His parents wanted him to be comfortable even though the prognosis was not the best. And I realised that even these little surgeries are huge moments for parents to see their children put under general anaesthesia. And the wait for them to come out may seem eternal. The title of this poem is sixteen hours but in reality it must feel like sixteen million hours...

# REAL LIFE SUPERHUMAN

This is real life
No cameras
No script
Just a reality
I never wanted

Look you think
It seems easy
To say I'm ok
When in fact
You don't see
The days when
I'm so out of it

The pain devours
What little fight
Left within me,
The mucositis
Is mean as the
Monsters under
My bed

You may say
I will get better
But empty promise
Is not in my interest
Bring out the guarantee,
Hath my health no warranty?

I watch people
Talking about struggles
On those big screens

But let's keep it real
Many of our stories
Are never told

Man I've travelled
This far I can't afford
To lose -
I've seen flat lines
But my life is not
Going to end flat

My cancer said
I'm not going to make it,
Pushing me hard
Testing my limits
But I'm not giving up
I will keep fighting

This is real life
This is real pain
Not an illusion but
I am superhuman
With all that
I've been through
I am not playing,
Just keeping it real.


**#Inspiration:**

This poem is dedicated to all the children fighting and facing your little battles every day. This was written in hope that you realise that your stories will not go unknown. Your struggles will pay off one day. Don't ever give up no matter how discouraged you may feel on days when you feel that you may not make it past that day. You will make it – yes you will. Power to all you fellow real life superhumans!

# LE PARADIS/GLORIOUS VICTORY

*J'ai trop souffert*
*Pendant ma vie*
*Mais un jour je crois*
*Que l'orage passera*
*Et on sera enfin libre*
*Pour fêter cette vie, ce paradis*
*Avec lequel on est béni*

Sun is rising finally
On the darkest horizon
Can you hear
A faint miracle
Awakening like
The morning glory
Blossoming in
The African desert

There is hope reborn
Again like a newborn
Fresh from the womb
After months of trials
Like new life
And a rebirth of faith
After a life of challenge
Overcoming struggles
To carry the victory
Of life home once more

The spirits cry
The cure is come!
The angels sing
A child has healed!
A wounded heart
Mends by sheer
Strength in
Self belief
Uplifting all around

*Le paradis*
*C'est pas loin d'ici*
*Pas besoin de chercher*
*Dans un autre monde*
*C'est juste ici*
*Dans ton cœur*
*Aie la foi en toi*

The day will come
When your glory
Is restored
And you will
Get a chance
To live life
All over again
A paradise
To cherish
A victory
To keep
Safe in the
Hands of hope

To restore
Faith and trust
In a soul once lost
Deep In the trenches
Of despondence

*Je sais que*
*Tu auras ce que*
*Tu veux et ce que*
*Tu cherches ta vie entière*
*Car le Bonne Dieu*
*Ne te quitteras jamais*
*Et te rassureras*
*Que tu vas toujours réussir !*

Do not look too far ahead
My friend the glory days
Are soon to come!

**#Inspiration:**

This poem is a fitting close to this compilation as it combines the best of both of my Anglophone and Francophone worlds which are equally close to my heart. It is filled with a powerful imagery and strong symbols of victory. Glory to all those who survived the battles and glory to those who have made history with their stories! Keep the fire of faith burning bright and the glory days are indeed soon to come, hang in there and stay strong everyone. Love, Pravin xx.

To: Dr Pravin.

Before saying that you are an extraordinary doctor,
i want to tell you that you are an extraordinary human.
being. Thanks for showing so much care and concern
towards my son condition during the stay.
Thanks for teaching me the different between Fact & Faith.
You always give strength to your patients to recover.
Thanks for your Sincerity, comcern and understanding.

You are truly a doctor.

From:
Your BFF
Red. 32. mmmmmm

At the end of this compilation, I wanted to share this note from a mother I received recently. Her child required a prolonged stay for a respiratory illness which improved gradually. Her message was so powerful and special that I decided to share it in this compilation as it truly embodies my wish, aim and purpose of doing what I am doing for the children. I hope it inspires everyone to know that sometimes there is a difference between fact and faith and we walk on the fine line in the middle as doctors who help to heal and who also help to bring comfort to our patients always. There is a humanity that we should never forget for it makes us feel a little more and care a little harder for our patients. (P.S. the drawing was the cutest bit, kudos to this mum for the lovely message & illustration!)

# MERCI

Thank you to everyone who has been so supportive of my paediatric palliative care and complex care dream and journey thus far. Thank you to Mum for being with me every step of the way. Thank you to the Paediatric Oncology, High Dependency/Intensive Care Unit & Neonatology Teams for all their support all the way – you mean so much to me. Of note, thank you to Dr Judith for the lovely foreword and for guiding me through my postings and residency, Dr Lee JH (guardian of my Mariah secret;)), Dr Siti, Dr Mervin, Dr Loh Lik Eng, Dr Mok for being every so kind and gracious to me during my high dependency and first intensive care posting ever. Thank you to Dr Soh, Dr Enrica, Dr Prasad, Prof Tan AM, Prof Tan Cheng Lim (my biggest fan of all time, thank you Prof!), Prof Chan MY, Dr Joyce, Dr Mya, Dr Khawn & Heidi for being such great supporters and fans of my poetry – I really appreciate it and I appreciate all of you for your meaningful work for all the patients you have touched with your hearts and hands. Thank you to my very special neonatology team for nurturing me & believing in me – Dr Amudha, Dr Pooja, Dr Alim, Dr Suresh, Dr Alvin, Dr Krishna, Dr Simrita, Dr Melissa, Dr Yee Yin, Dr Eleah, Dr Genevieve, Dr Janlie, Dr Maria & everyone else who works so hard to keep the babies alive and well, blessed to have rotated with you. Thank you to all the special people I have worked with across the various postings (the spectrum is incredible & seeing the patients & families makes it all worth it!) – Dr Esther (miss you!), Dr Chong SL, Dr Ng YH, Dr Indra, Dr Veena L, Dr Christina O, Dr Chiou FK, Prof Phua KB, Prof Tan TH, Dr J.Choo, Dr Monika (& the cardio techs Kim, XinYi & team), Dr Tan ES, Dr Ting TW, Dr Saumya, Breanna (I felt we woulda been best friends in school, dedicating the poem P.K.U to you!) for being very patient and always willing to spare an extra moment to share your knowledge with all of us. Thank you to the Paediatric Anaesthesia Department for taking me under your wing during my elective. Many thanks to Dr Angela Y, Dr Angela T, Dr Sharon, the anaesthesia residents & team.

A special thanks to the seniors who have been such great friends, fans and teachers through it all – Prof Chay OM, Dr Joel C, Dr Natalie, Dr Lynette Wee, Dr Rashida, Sin Wee (gurl that sense of fashion and my new bestie!), my fans Theresa T & Alicia, Samantha (keepin it fierce & real with that eye makeup, please teach me!), Ka$hfi (moneymaker, love you), Lynette Goh, Shi Yun, Joyce Tan, Daniel Chan (my big brother since forever!), Pippa, Wing Yee, Dr Lay Ong (the iron tinman from Oz with a heart) & Katrina. And shout out to my dear friends for carrying me thru rough times & pushin me through all the way (& for the laughs, after all laughter *IS* le best medicine!) – Christopher (man where do I begin?), Anu, Devaki, Sheau Yun, Misa, Janine, Jia Min, Priya, Mei Ching, Kwan Rui, Peachy, Debbie, Y.Zhi Min, Yuqini, Chester HJ, Sam Q, Maria, Riza, Jocelyn, Rushcelle, Janelle, Aubrey and my Filipina community ♥ To the fans from way back when – KenChin, Nams, Colin Ng, Ying Tai, Ian Loh, Evan, Zi Hao, Tri, Lulu, Hester, Aimee, WeiQi, Jean, Charissa, Aliviya, Theresa (merci pour les cartes postales!), Cammie, Nish, Prof Tay Sook Muay & Catherine Lim (your stories are phenomenal!). To my lovely Star PALS fam, Dr Chong PH, Serene, Kay, Geraldine, Mel B – you're my daily inspiration. To the inpatient palliative team, Dr Komal T & Dr Wynn, thank you for your hard work. Rohanna, Salve & all the staff of KK who work so hard for us every day – you know I can't thank you enough xoxo. To the French fam – vous me manquez bcp (Clarisse, Sébastian, Sandy, Jabeen, Dr Annie, Dr Ghaidaa, Dr Santana, Natalie Aubin – je reviendrai un jour). And of course to the English teacher who started it all...Mdm Marjorie Tan, this one's for you! Last but not least, to all the children and their families past, present & future, may this anthology serve as a reminder that you will always be in our memories, our hearts & our prayers. Peace & Love always, Pravin – you're never alone xx.

**Other Authorhouse Titles by R.R.Pravin:**

**Paediatric Palliative Care/Complex Care Anthologies**

Caught in the Mo(u)rning Rain (2014)
Dreamcatcher : Le Capteur de Rêves (2015)
Do they have telephones up in heaven? (2017)
Fire, Faith & Glory (2018)

**Novels**

African Girl (2008)
When Angels Bleed & Devils Lie (2009)
Phantom of Keys (2011)
Eyes of A Broken Warrior & Other Short Stories (2013)
The Good Girl's Guide to Mean Boys (2016)

**Poetry**

Country Soul & Caravan Magic ; *Un Séjour à Strasbourg* (2018)

**Collaborations:**
Heartfelt: A Compilation of Short Stories (Yong Loo Lin School of Medicine 2013)
Timba's Rainbow Journey (English Corner Publishers Singapore 2013)
Will's Magical Christmas (English Corner Publishers Singapore 2013)

**Website:** https://www.facebook.com/palliativecareforchildren

Lightning Source UK Ltd.
Milton Keynes UK
UKHW01n1326280818
327922UK00002B/16/P